HEART FAILURE AND RHEUMATIC FEVER

Your Ideal Medical Study Companion

ISHMAEL ONSERIO

Copyright © 2020 by Ishmael Onserio
All rights reserved.

This book or any portion thereof may not be reproduced or used in any such manner whatsoever without written permission of the publisher except in the case of brief quotations in the context of book reviews.

First Published on, February 2020

ISBN: 9798612346036

Published By
Amazon Publishing Company © 1996-2020, Amazon.com, Inc. or its affiliates Website: www.amazon.com

Printed in the United States of America

DEDICATION

This book is dedicated to Mr. Fred Momanyi Nyambeche, my senior school level principal. His foundations on real education have been a totem in my life.

To Hannah Kegwaro, my elementary school instructor. Your love and passion to teach will always be remembered. May god grant her peace and healing.

To all survivors of rheumatic fever, especially those with rheumatic heart disease. Recovery is on your way.

CONTENTS

Dedication	*iii*
Contents	*iv*
Acknowledgement	*v*
Abbreviations	*vi*
Preface	*ix*
Heart Failure	*1*
Rheumatic Fever	*46*
References	*67*

ACKNOWLEDGMENTS

First and foremost, I thank God, the Almighty, for His blessings throughout my life and especially on this art of writing.
I would like to express my deep and sincere gratitude to my brother, Tim for his moral, physical and academic support; his love and motivation have deeply inspired me.
I am extending my heartfelt gratitude to my Mum and Dad, for their unwavering prayers, love and sacrifices. With God's grace they have kept me going.
Also, I express my thanks to my sisters, brothers and our family at large for their support and valuable prayers. Blessings.

~

ABBREVIATIONS

ABG: Arterial Blood Gas

BNP: B-type Natriuretic Peptide

ACC: American College of Cardiology

ACE: Angiotensin Converting Enzyme

ADH: Anti-Diuretic Hormone

ADHF: Acute Decompensated Heart Failure

AF: Atrial Fibrillation

AHA: American Heart Association

ANP: Atrial Natriuretic Peptide

ARBs: Angiotensin II Receptor Blockers

BCE: Before the Common Era (Before the Current Era)

CAD: Coronary Artery Disease

CHF/D: Congestive Heart Failure/Disease

CNS: Central Nervous System

CO: Cardiac Output

COPD: Chronic Obstructive Pulmonary Disease

CPAP: Continuous Positive Airway Pressure

CRT: Cardiac Resynchronization Therapy

CS: Cardio-Renal Syndrome

CT: Computed Tomography

EDV: End-Diastolic Volume

ECG: Electrocardiogram

EF: Ejection Fraction

FBC: Full Blood Count

GFR: Glomerular Filtration Rate

HCC: Hepatocellular Carcinoma

HF: Heart Failure

HR: Heart Rate
HTN: Hypertension
IHD: Ischemic Heart Disease
IE: Infective Endocarditis
IV: Intravenous
JVP: Jugular Venous Pressure
LFTs: Liver Functions Tests
LSHF: Left-Sided Heart Failure
LVEF: Left Ventricular Ejection Fraction
MI: Myocardial Infarction
MRI: Magnetic Resonance Imaging
NYHA: New York Heart Association
PA: Posterior Anterior
RAAS: Renin–Angiotensin–Aldosterone System
RFTs: Renal Functions Tests
RHD: Rheumatic Heart Disease
RSHF: Right-Sided Heart Failure
RVH: Right Ventricular Hypertrophy
SV: Stroke Volume
TFTs: Thyroid Functions Tests
TPR: Temperature, Pulse and Respiration
VT: Ventricular Fibrillation

~

"Prayer is not asking. It is a longing of the soul. It is daily admission of one's weakness. It is better in prayer to have a heart without words than words without a heart."

∾ **Mahatma Gandhi**

PREFACE

The human heart is one of the most important organs in the entire human body. It is really nothing more than a pump that is composed of muscles which pump blood throughout the entire body, beating approximately 72 times per minute of our lives.

The heart pumps blood, which carries all the vital materials which help our bodies function and removes the waste products that we do not need. For example, the brain requires oxygen and glucose, which, if not received continuously, will cause it to lose consciousness.

Muscles and glands need sufficient supplies of raw materials (oxygen and nutrients) from which to manufacture the specific secretions. If the heart ever ceases to pump blood the body begins to shut down and after a very short period of time it dies.

On the other hand, the immune system is a vast network of cells and tissues which is constantly on the lookout for invaders, and once an enemy is spotted, a complex attack is mounted. Without an immune system, our bodies would be open to attack from bacteria, viruses, parasites, and many more. It is the immune system that keeps the body healthy as it drifts through a sea of pathogens.

This book goes beyond the ordinary to elaborate clearly on the two conditions that affect these two systems (Heart Failure and Rheumatic Fever). It makes these two conditions well understood with one time reading. The book goes into an extra mile to explain their management in a well elaborated manner.

1
~ HEART FAILURE ~

AN OVERVIEW OF THE ANATOMY AND PHYSIOLOGY OF THE HEART

The human heart is a muscular organ that pumps blood to all various parts of the body. This mechanism is achieved through a collaboration of functionally unified structures including the heart itself and the blood vessels (arteries, capillaries and veins).

The human has four chambers, the *two upper chambers (atria)* joining to the *two lower chambers (ventricles)*. An internal partition separates the left chambers from the right ones and is called the *septum*. It prevents the *oxygenated* blood from mixing with *deoxygenated* blood. The atria and ventricles from each side are separated from each other by a bunch of flaps called valves.

The atria receive blood that is returning to the heart from the two routes of the circulation system. This blood is then channeled into ventricles that pumps the blood. The right atrium receives deoxygenated blood from body circulation while the left atrium receives oxygenated blood from the pulmonary circulation, specifically from the lungs.

The right ventricle pumps deoxygenated blood out of the heart through the pulmonary artery to the lungs, while the left ventricle pumps blood out of the heart to the rest of the body tissues through the aorta. The left ventricular muscle wall is thicker than that of the right, as pumping blood to the lungs is a relatively easier

§ Heart Failure §

work compared to pumping of it to all parts of the body.

Blood circulates through the chambers of the heart in a well-defined system. The right ventricle pumps blood out of the heart to the lungs, where it picks up oxygen. Blood then returns from the lungs and flows into the left atrium and then into the left ventricle, which pumps it back out into the rest of the body tissues. This blood finally returns to the heart, flowing into the right atrium through superior and inferior venacava.

One-way valves between the heart's chambers keep the blood cycling through the heart in the right direction. The valves have flaps, called cusps, which open when blood is pumped through them and snap shut to prevent back-flow. The mitral valve separates the left atrium from the left ventricle and the tricuspid valve does the same on the right side of the heart. Theses valves are also called right or left atrioventricular valves depending on which side of the heart they lie.

The cycle of blood circulation in the body occurs in two phases. The first one is diastole (a period when the ventricles relax to allow blood to flow into them from the atria). The other one is systole (a period when the ventricles contract and eject blood into the aorta and pulmonary artery). These phases altogether are referred to as a cardiac cycle, or heartbeat.

The heart weighs around 350g and is roughly the size of an adult's clenched fist. It is enclosed in the mediastinal cavity of the thorax between the lungs and extends downwards to the left

§ Heart Failure §

between the second and fifth intercostal space.

The heart has a middle muscular layer, the myocardium, which is made up of cardiac muscle cells, and an inner lining is called the endocardium.

The heart is enclosed in a sac, the pericardium, which protects it and prevents it from over-expanding, anchoring it inside the thorax. The pericardium is attached to the diaphragm and inner surface of the sternum, and is made up of:

- The *fibrous pericardium*, composed of a loosely fitting but dense layer of connective tissue
- The *serous pericardium* or epicardium, composed of the parietal and visceral layers
- A *film of serous fluid* between the fibrous and serous pericardium that allows them to glide smoothly against each other.

§ Heart Failure §

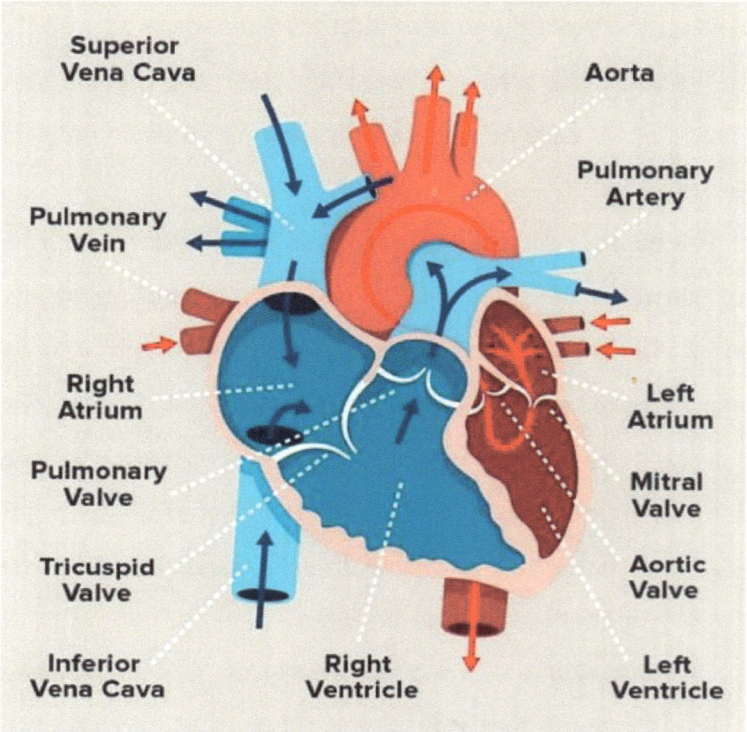

The Structure of the Heart

Heart Pumping Mechanisms

Various physical measures are usually employed when assessing how well the heart is working. These include cardiac output, stroke volume and the ejection fraction.

The heart pumping mechanism is determined by the following basic components:

<u>*Cardiac Output*</u>: This is the volume of blood the heart pumps through the circulatory system in one minute.

Cardiac output (CO) = Stroke Volume (SV) x Heart Rate (HR)

§ Heart Failure §

Ejection Fraction: This is the fraction of blood pumped out of the heart by ventricles with each heartbeat.

Ejection fraction = stroke volume ÷ end-diastolic volume

"Ejection" refers to the amount of blood that is pumped out of the heart's main pumping chamber during each heartbeat and *"Fraction"* refers to the fact that, even in a healthy heart, some blood always remains within this chamber after each heartbeat.

Stroke Volume: It is the volume of blood pumped out by the left ventricle in one heartbeat.

Stroke volume = end-diastolic volume - end-systolic volume

Stroke volume is determined by:

- *Preload:* This is the volume of blood entering the right ventricle at end of diastole. It depends on venous return and compliance. Preload increases with fluid volume build up and vasoconstriction ("squeezes" blood from vascular system into heart). Preload decreases with fluid volume losses and vasodilatation (able to "hold" more blood, therefore less returning to heart).

- *Afterload:* It is the force needed to eject blood into circulation from the left ventricle. It depends upon arterial blood pressure, pulmonary arterial pressure and the status of the heart valves such as valvular heart disease increases afterload. It also increases with hypertension and vasoconstriction. Afterload decreased with vasodilatation.

§ Heart Failure §

> *Myocardial Contractility/Inotropy:* This is the force of muscular contractions. Contractility increases with sympathetic stimulation (effects of epinephrine), positive inotropes (medications that increase contractility, such as digoxin, sympathomimetics).

Contractility decreases with infarcted tissue; no contractile strength, ischemic tissue, reduced contractile strength, electrolyte/acid-base imbalance, negative inotropes (medications that decrease contractility, such as beta blockers).

In a healthy adult, the normal range for cardiac output is 4 L/minute to 8 L/minute, the stroke volume will be between 55 mL and 100 mL, and the ejection fraction is between 55% and 70%.

HEART FAILURE

Heart failure is a clinical syndrome that results from any structural or functional cardiac disorder that impairs the ability of ventricles to fill with or eject blood effectively. It is the pathophysiological process in which the heart as a pump is unable to meet metabolic requirements (oxygen and substrates) of the body tissues despite the body's venous is either normal or increased.

Heart failure is a clinical syndrome that results from the inability of the heart to maintain adequate circulation. It is a progressive disorder associated with high morbidity and mortality. Its prognosis

§ Heart Failure §

is generally poor; approximately 50% die within five years.

Heart failure is often referred as Congestive Heart Failure/Disease (CHF/D). While this condition is often referred to simply as "Heart Failure," CHF specifically refers to the stage in which fluid builds up around the heart and making the pumping mechanisms inefficient.

Additionally, the term congestive heart failure is normally used when there is failure of both heart ventricles (the most common). This eventually leads to blood and other fluids pooling in various organs and regions of the body such as lungs, abdomen, liver and lower body extremities.

Therefore, this condition comes as a result of two heart malfunctions:

- *Systolic Dysfunctions*: This occurs when the left ventricle fails to contract normally leading to reduced muscle force to push blood into the circulatory system. This force makes the heart to pump properly.

- *Diastolic Dysfunctions*: This is also called diastolic failure and it happens when the muscles of the left ventricle become so stiff; they can no longer relax and therefore the heart can't quite fill with blood during the diastolic cycles.

§ Heart Failure §

EPIDEMIOLOGY OF HEART FAILURE

Heart failure has been known since ancient times with the Ebers papyrus commenting on it around 1550 BCE.

Heart failure is a common, costly, and potentially fatal condition. In 2015 it affected about 40 million people globally.

Overall around 2% of adults have heart failure and in those over the age of 65, this increases to 6–10%. Rates are predicted to increase.

The risk of death is about 35% the first year after diagnosis; while by the second year the risk of death is less than 10% for those who remain alive. This degree of risk of death is similar to some cancers.

More than 20 million people have heart failure worldwide. Prevalence of heart failure in India due to coronary heart disease, hypertension, obesity, diabetes and rheumatic heart disease to range from 1.3 to 4.6 million, with an annual incidence of 491 600-1.8 million.

Heart failure is the leading cause of hospitalization in people older than 65 years. 1–2% of the population (About 5.7 million individuals in the US have heart failure).

The incidence is higher among African Americans, Hispanics, and Native Americans. Increases with age; about 10% of individuals > 60 years old are affected. Systolic heart disease is the most common form of HF overall.

In the United Kingdom, the disease is the reason for 5% of

§ Heart Failure §

emergency hospital admissions.

CAUSES OF HEART FAILURE
Summary of the Causes
To easily remember the various causes of heart failure always remember the mnemonic **FAILURE:**

Faulty heart valves
AV and SL valve problems (due to congenital issues or infection (endocarditis) that causes blood to back flow (regurgitation) or stenosis (narrowing of the valves that increases pressure of blood flow through the valves). This causes the heart to work harder and become weak over time.

Arrhythmias
Atrial fibrillation or tachycardia.

Myocardial infarction
Coronary artery disease: part of the heart muscle dies due to a blockage in the coronary arteries; muscle become ischemic and can die (main cause of left ventricular systolic dysfunction).

Lineage (congenital)
Family history

Uncontrolled Hypertension
Overtime this can lead to stiffening of the heart walls because with untreated HTN the heart has to work harder and this causes the ventricles to become stiff.

§ Heart Failure §

Recreational Drug

Use (cocaine) or alcohol abuse.

Envaders *(instead of Invaders)*

Viruses or infections that attack the heart muscle.

Description of the Causes of Heart Failure

The above immediate sub-unit describes the easier way to remember the main causes of HF. The following are the general causes of heart failure:

Vascular

These are the most common causes of heart failure:

- *Ischemic heart disease (35-40%):* infarction causes impaired ventricular function, therefore reduced contractility function and HF. IHD are the most common cause of HF along with HTN.

- *Hypertension (15-20%):* increases strain on the heart, since the heart has to pump blood against a high afterload, leading to hypertrophy which increase the chances of arrhythmias. The heart would eventually get too big for the coronary system to perfuse leading to IHD and compromised ventricular function.

Muscular

Cardiomyopathy is a common cause of heart failure under this group. Dilated cardiomyopathies are often idiopathic. It is the disease of the heart muscles that is not secondary to IHD, HTN, and

§ Heart Failure §

valvular, congenital or pericardial disease. It has several types:

- *Congestive:* weakening and dilation of ventricular walls leading to overstretching therefore reduced contractile efficiency. Is the most common cause of HF in the absence of IHD, valvular disease and HTN; this might have a familial link.
- *Restrictive:* this is the reduced heart compliance without significant increase in muscle wall thickness leading to reduced EDV and CO. It's brought by sarcoidosis, amyloidosis, hemochromatosis and endocardial fibrosis.
- Dilated cardiomyopathy (30%).
- *Hypertrophic cardiomyopathy:* it is the thickening of the heart muscle wall leading to reduced compliance and therefore reduced CO. The thickening involves an increase in fibrous tissue of the heart, which increases the chances of arrhythmias such as ventricular fibrillation, which is a common cause of death in young adults. This disease has a strong familial link.
- Congenital heart disease.

Valvular

Valvular heart disease may lead to either acute or chronic heart failure:

- Stenotic valves
- Regurgitant valves

§ Heart Failure §

Electrical

Arrhythmias (abnormalities of normal conduction) may cause acute heart failure through decompensation. These includes:

- *Bradycardia:* CO = HR X SV. Therefore, reduced HR reduces CO.
- *Tachycardia:* Reduced ventricular filling duration, increased heart oxygen demand and ventricular dilatation.
- *Abnormal atrial and ventricular contractions:* AF removes active ventricular filling leading to reduced EDV and CO. VT also causes reduced EDV due to reduced ventricular filling period.

High output

Typically, heart failure is caused by a reduced cardiac output. In some cases, however, the cardiac output may be raised but the systemic vascular resistance be very low. Causes here include:

- Anaemia
- Septicemia due to toxic effects of infection on heart itself along with vasodilation and tachycardia increase myocardial oxygen demand. Patients with chronic HF are more susceptible to infections.
- Thyrotoxicosis
- Liver failure

Alcohol

Acute heart failure, arrhythmias such as AF and dilated cardiomyopathy in alcoholics.

§ Heart Failure §

Myxedema

This can cause HF due to direct effects on the myocardium, bradycardia and pericardial disease.

COMPENSATORY MECHANISMS

These mechanisms attempt to maintain sufficient blood pressure to perfuse vital organs by compensating for the decrease in cardiac output that occurs in heart failure.

The Frank-Starling mechanism

Frank-Starling relationship to this indicates that ventricular output increases in relation to preload, i.e. with a greater stretch of myocardial fibers (larger diastolic volume); there will be a greater force of contraction generated. In heart failure, a decreased stroke volume results in reduced chamber emptying, with higher than normal diastolic volume.

This induces a greater stroke volume for the subsequent contraction to help empty the ventricle and preserve forward cardiac output.

However, this mechanism has limits, and at markedly elevated diastolic volumes, the stretch of myofibers becomes too great and suboptimal for generating a strong contraction.

Myocardial Hypertrophy

Wall stress is often increased in heart failure due to either ventricular dilatation or the need to generate high systolic pressures to overcome excessive afterload.

Wall stress is estimated from Laplace's relationship, in which the wall stress (σ) is proportional to ventricular pressure (P) and ventricular chamber radius (r), and inversely proportional to ventricular wall thickness (h).

In response to a sustained increase in pressure and chamber radius, hypertrophy of the ventricular myocytes is stimulated. The increased mass of muscle fibers serves to maintain contractile force and counteract the elevated ventricular wall stress.

Eventually, the chamber may dilate out of proportion to wall thickness, resulting in excessive hemodynamic burden on the contractile units, rapid deterioration of ventricular function and worsening of symptomatology. Lowering wall stress as a way to slow the remodeling process is a common therapeutic target.

Neuro-Hormonal Mechanisms

In the early stages of heart failure, these mechanisms help maintain a near normal perfusion to vital organs by increasing systemic vascular resistance as a way to balance the fall in cardiac output (blood pressure (BP) = cardiac output (CO) × total peripheral resistance (TPR)).

In addition, activation of neuro-hormonal mechanisms leads to salt and water retention with a consequent increase in intravascular volume and preload, which maximizes stroke volume via the Frank-

§ Heart Failure §

Starling mechanism.

Renin-Angiotensin-Aldosterone System (RAAS): The pathway leads to the activation of angiotensin II and has the following effects:

Angiotensin II: Leads to vasoconstriction: Increases TPR to maintain BP. Increased intravascular volume to increase preload to raise the SV via Frank-Starling mechanism. Angiotensin II does this by:

- Stimulating thirst at hypothalamus
- Increasing aldosterone secretion at adrenal cortex.

Aldosterone: Increased water retention via increased sodium resorption. This increases preload, in turn increasing the SV.

Antidiuretic Hormone (ADH or Vasopressin): Increased secretion thought to be induced by arterial baroreceptors (detecting decreased CO) and increased angiotensin II levels. Promotes water retention in the distal collecting tubule, in order to increase preload.

Adrenergic Nervous System

Decreased CO results in decreased perfusion pressure sensed by baroreceptors in carotid sinus and the aortic arch. Central and peripheral chemoreflex activation induces epinephrine, norepinephrine, and vasopressin release. This results in an increased sympathetic outflow to heart and peripheral circulation and decreased parasympathetic tone.

§ Heart Failure §

- Increased HR and contractility directly increase cardiac output (CO = HR × SV)
- Peripheral vasoconstriction
- Venous Increases preload (venous return)
- Arteriolar raises peripheral vascular resistance, to maintain BP.

Unfortunately, despite these compensatory mechanisms, there is progressive decline in the heart's ability to contract and relax in the face of persistent hemodynamic challenges.

Furthermore, chronic activation of the above mechanisms ultimately becomes maladaptive and induces further worsening of cardiac performance.

Serious Consequences of Compensatory Mechanisms

Continuous sympathetic activation results in down regulation of β-adrenergic receptors with decreased sensitivity to circulating catecholamines and less inotropic response.

Increased heart rate augments metabolic demands and can further reduce performance by increasing myocardial cell death.

Increased circulating volume and preload ultimately overwhelm Frank-Starling mechanism and heart's ability to maintain forward flow, resulting in worsening of lung vasculature congestion.

Increased total peripheral resistance results in higher afterload, impeding the left ventricle's stroke volume and reducing cardiac output.

Chronically elevated angiotensin II and aldosterone trigger production of cytokines, which activate macrophages and stimulate fibroblasts resulting in adverse heart remodeling.

N/B: All organs (liver, lungs, legs, etc.) return blood to heart. When heart begins to fail/ weaken it becomes unable to pump blood forward and fluid backs up and this increases pressure within all organs.

Organ Response

LUNGS: They become congested and there is increased effort to breathe. Fluid starts to escape into alveoli (pulmonary edema). The fluid interferes with O2 exchange (hypoxia) and this aggravates shortness of breath; shortness of breath during exertion may be early symptoms progress where later may require extra pillows at night to breathe (orthopnea) and experience "P.N.D." or paroxysmal nocturnal dyspnea.

LEGS, ANKLES, FEET: LEGS, ANKLES, FEET: blood from feet and legs back-up of fluid and pressure in these areas, as heart unable to pump blood as promptly as received increase fluid within feet and legs (pedal/dependent edema) and increase in weight.

TYPES AND CLASSIFICATION OF HEART FAILURE

There are many types of HF. This book has covered them in the writer's format to bring out the clear distinction between these

§ Heart Failure §

kinds. They are as follows:

a) Systolic and Diastolic Systolic HF

The systolic type is described as the inability of the heart to contract efficiently to eject adequate volumes of blood to meet the body metabolic demand (the most common type). It is characterized by reduced left ventricular ejection fraction (LVEF); the heart is pumping out a reduced proportion of the blood that fills its ventricles during diastole. This results in ventricular dilatation and characteristic eccentric remodeling.

Diastolic HF is characterized by impaired ventricular relaxation or filling. Contraction is unaffected and as such the LVEF is preserved. Diastolic heart failure may be called 'heart failure with preserved LVEF'. Ventricular hypertrophy tends to develop, and characteristic concentric remodeling may occur. It is the reduction in the heart compliance resulting in compromised ventricular filling and therefore ejection (e.g. in pericardial disease, restrictive cardiomyopathy, tamponade).

Cardiac remodeling refers to changes in cardiac size; shape and function in response to cardiac injury or increased load (e.g. exercise). Pathological remodeling may occur after conditions such as myocardial infarction or cardiomyopathy.

b) Low output and high output HF

Low-output HF is a type of heart failure resulting from reduced

§ Heart Failure §

cardiac output (Most common). *High-output HF* is a type of heart failure that occurs in normal or high cardiac output due to metabolic demand and supply mismatch, either due to reduced blood oxygen carrying capacity (Anemia) or increase body metabolic demand (thyrotoxicosis).

c) Acute and chronic heart failure

Acute HF is a type of HF that presents with an acute onset of symptom presentation usually due to an acute event such as MI, persistent arrhythmia, mechanical event (ruptured valve, ventricular aneurysm).

Chronic HF on the other hand is a type comes with a slow symptom presentation usually due to slow progressive underlying disease e.g. CAD, HTN among others.

Acute-on-chronic HF is an acute deterioration of a chronic condition, usually following an acute event e.g. anemia, infections, arrhythmias or MI.

d) Right and left sided HF

Because the two ventricles of the heart represent two separate pumping systems, it is possible for one to fail alone for a short period.

Left HF is characterized by the inability of the left ventricle to pump adequate amount of blood leading to pulmonary circulation congestion and pulmonary edema. Usually results in RHF due to pulmonary hypertension.

Right HF presents with the inability of the right ventricle to pump adequate amount of blood leading to systemic venous congestion, therefore peripheral edema and hepatic congestion and tenderness.

e) Forward and backward heart failure

Forward heart failure results from inadequate discharge of blood into arterial system leading to poor tissue perfusion and excess Na+ reabsorption through RAAS.

Backward heart failure results from failure of one or both ventricles to fill normally and discharge its contents, causing back pressure on the atria and venous system.

RIGHT-SIDED HEART FAILURE

The right ventricle fails as effective pump. The right ventricle cannot eject blood returning through vena cavae. Blood therefore backs up into systemic circulation.

There is an increased pressure in systemic capillaries forces fluid out of capillaries into interstitial spaces leading to tissue edema. It also called Cor Pulmonale.

It usually occurs as a result of left heart failure. The right ventricle pumps blood to the lungs for oxygen. Occasionally isolated right heart failure can occur due to lung disease or blood clots to the lung (pulmonary embolism).

Right-sided heart failure causes congestion of blood in the

§ Heart Failure §

heart and this increases the pressure in the inferior vena cava (which normally brings "used" blood back to the heart for reoxygenation). This built-up pressure causes the hepatic veins to become very congested with blood which leads to hepatomegaly and swelling peripherally.

Right-sided heart failure is usually caused from left-sided heart failure because of the increased fluid pressure backing up from the left side to the right. This causes the right side of the heart to become overworked. Other causes include pulmonary heart disease *"Cor Pulmonale"* as a complication from pulmonary hypertension or COPD.

Signs and Symptoms of RSHF

Remember the mnemonic **SWELLING** when figuring out how the RSHF presents (fluid is backing up in the right side of the heart which causes fluid to back-up in the hepatic veins and peripheral veins). Its features include the following:

- **S**welling of legs, hands, liver, abdomen
- **W**eight gain
- **E**dema (pitting)
- **L**arge neck veins (jugular venous distention)
- **L**ethargic (weak and very tired)
- **I**rregular heart rate (atrial fibrillation)
- *Nocturia (frequent urination at night):* Lying down elevates the legs and allows the extra fluid to enter into

the vascular system which allows the kidneys to eliminate the extra fluid.
- Girth of abdomen increased (from swelling of the liver and building up fluid in the abdomen), can't breathe well and this causes nausea and anorexia.

LEFT SIDED HEART FAILURE

The left side of the heart cannot pump blood out of the heart efficiently, so blood starts to back up in the lungs.

It is the most common type of heart failure. Left-sided heart failure is likely to lead to right sided heart failure.

In left sided heart failure, left ventricle cardiac output is less then volume received from pulmonary circulation; blood accumulates in the left ventricle, left atrium.

Pulmonary congestion forcing fluid from pulmonary capillaries into pulmonary tissue and alveoli causing pulmonary interstitial edema and impaired gas exchange.

The left ventricle becomes too weak and unable to squeeze blood out properly; this heart failure can be either systolic or diastolic.

Systolic: In left ventricular systolic dysfunction, remember systolic is the contraction or "squeezing" phase of the heart. In systolic dysfunction, there is an issue with the left ventricle being able to eject blood properly out of the ventricle and the organs can't get all that rich oxygenated blood it just received from the

§ Heart Failure §

lungs. Patients will have a low ejection fraction.

What is ejection fraction? Ejection fraction is a calculation used to determine the severity of heart failure on the left side. A normal EF is 50% or greater meaning that more than half of the blood that fills inside the ventricles is being pumped out. An EF can be measured with an echocardiogram or nuclear stress test. An EF of 40% or less is a diagnosis for heart failure.

Diastolic: In left ventricular diastolic dysfunction, remember diastole is the filling or resting phase of the heart. In diastolic dysfunction, the ventricle is too stiff to allow for normal filling of blood. Since there isn't an issue with contraction but filling the ejection fraction is usually normal.

Signs and Symptoms of LSHF

In this type remember the mnemonic **DROWNING** (these patients are literally drowning in their own fluid from the heart's failure to pump efficiently). Features include the following:

Difficulty breathing: This is due to increased pulmonary capillary oncotic pressure from left-sided backflow causes extravasation of fluid into the pulmonary interstitium, which then leads to reduced pulmonary compliance and increased airway resistance. There is also an increased ventilatory drive secondary to hypoxemia, a consequence of increased pulmonary capillary pressures and ventilation/perfusion mismatch due to inadequate CO.

§ Heart Failure §

Rales (crackles): Opening of small airways that were closed by interstitial edema prior to inspiration; initially present at lung bases where hydrostatic forces are greatest, but worsening pulmonary edema is associated with crackles in higher lung fields.

Orthopnea (cannot tolerate lying down; must sit-up to breath, especially while sleeping): There is redistribution of extravascular fluid from the periphery into dependent areas when supine (i.e. lungs) exacerbates dyspnea as the ventricles cannot adapt to the acute increase in volume; this results in increased pulmonary capillary pressure and worsening of interstitial pulmonary edema.

Weakness (extremely tired and fatigued due to shortness of breath and heart can't compensate for increased activity): Nocturnal Paroxysmal dyspnea (awaking during sleep with extreme dyspnea).

Increased heart rate (due to fluid overload and the heart is trying to get the blood to organs but it can't because of muscle failure).

Nagging cough (can be frothy or blood-tinged sputum from fluid overload in the lungs; very bad sign). Caused by pulmonary congestion. Rupture of engorged bronchial veins can lead to hemoptysis.

Gaining weight from the body retaining fluid; 2 to 3 lbs. in a day or 5 lbs. in a week.

§ Heart Failure §

DIAGNOSIS OF HEART FAILURE

Classification and staging of HF help in making the correct diagnosis of the condition. This is done in relation to the features the patient presents with. These classifications indicate the severity of the failure. There are two major classification systems used to approach this. They are as follows:

- *American Heart Association/American College of Cardiology (AHA/ACC)*: These are stages of heart failure. Stages - progress in one direction due to cardiac remodeling.
- *New York Heart Association (NYHA):* This is the functional classifications, NYHA Classes: shift back/forth in individual patient (in response to Rx and/or progression of disease).

NYHA Functional Classification

The NYHA (New York Heart Association) functional classification system assesses the patient's functional capacities (i.e., limitations of physical activity and symptoms) and has prognostic value. NYHA class Characteristics are as follows:

- *Class I:* No limitations of physical activity; no symptoms of HF.
- *Class II:* Slight limitations of moderate or prolonged physical activity (e.g., symptoms after climbing 2 flights of stairs or heavy lifting); comfortable at rest.
- *Class III:* Marked limitations of physical activity (symptoms during daily activities like dressing, walking across rooms);

comfortable only at rest.
- *Class IV:* Confined to bed, discomfort during any form of physical activity; symptoms present at rest.

American Heart Association (AHA) Classification (2013)

The AHA classification system classifies patients according to their stage of the disease. It involves objective findings (patient history, diagnostic findings) as well as symptoms of HF. Stages and Objective Assessment Corresponding NYHA of AHA include the following:

- *Stage A:* At a high risk of HF but without structural heart disease.
- *Stage B:* Structural heart disease without signs or symptoms of HF
- *Stage C:* Structural heart disease with prior HF or current HF
- *Stage D:* Refractory HF requiring special interventions.

More Diagnostic Tests

The Framingham Criteria

This is a formal set of diagnostic criteria for congestive heart failure (CHF) that resulted from the well-known Framingham Heart Study (an excellent example of a prospective study, to be mentioned in any public health examinations!).

As with other diagnostic criteria systems this one makes use of *Major* and *Minor criteria* which are an important study aid in

§ Heart Failure §

themselves.

Diagnosis of congestive heart failure using the Framingham criteria requires simultaneous presence of 2 Major or 1 Major and 2 Minor criteria, which provide for a 100% sensitivity (but 78% specificity) value when diagnosing the symptoms and signs of CHF. The *major criteria* include the following diagnostic characteristics. They include:

- S3 heart sound present ('gallop' sound)
- Acute pulmonary oedema (left side of heart is unable to clear fluid from lungs).
- Weight loss of more than 4.5kg in 5 days when treated (patients lose their retained fluids).
- Paroxysmal nocturnal dyspnea
- Abdomino-jugular reflux (JVP waveform rises when pressure applied over liver area).
- Neck vein distended (i.e. JVP elevated at rest).
- Increased cardiac shadow on X-ray (cardiomegaly: heart occupies more than ≈50% of chest diameter).
- Crackles heard in lungs.

Minor criteria include the following defining characteristics:

- Hepatomegaly
- Pleural effusion
- Ankle oedema bilaterally
- Exertional dyspnoea
- Tachycardia

§ Heart Failure §

- Vital capacity decreased by a third of maximum value
- Nocturnal cough

The Minor criteria can only be used if they are not attributable to other medical conditions (e.g. pleural effusions cannot be due to infection, malignancy e.t.c).

CXR

This may show several changes depending on the severity of the heart failure such as Cardiomegaly (CTR (cardiothoracic ratio) >50% on PA, L or RVH, Pericardial effusion if cardiac silhouette has a globular appearance.

ECG

This may indicate the underlying cause of the heart failure such as:

- Myocardial infarction/ischemia
- Bundle Branch Block
- Ventricular hypertrophy
- Pericardial disease
- Arrhythmias

BNP (b-type Natriuretic Peptide) Blood Test

This is a biomarker released by the ventricles when there is excessive pressure in the heart due to its failure:

- <100 pg/mL no failure
- 100-300 pg/mL present
- 300 pg/mL mild

§ Heart Failure §

- 600 pg/mL moderate
- 900 pg/mL severe

Blood Tests

They are done to detect any underlying causes and the severity of the disease. Tests to determine the following are important:

- Anemia
- Hyponatremia (in severe disease due to dilution)
- Hypokalemia/Hyperkalemia
- LFT's to detect extent of liver congestion/damage
- RFT's to detect the severity of the disease (Inc. creatinine/urea).
- TFT's to rule out thyrotoxicosis or myxedema.

Echocardiogram

This is the only sensitive, non-invasive investigation that can confirm HF by detecting the ejection fraction, ventricular wall thickness and cardiac kinetics. Can also be used to detect underlying causes such as valvular diseases.

Angiography

This can be used to assess the extent of IHD.

Pulmonary Function Tests

It is important in excluding lung disease causing breathlessness.

§ Heart Failure §

Atrial Natriuretic Peptide (ANP)

Released when atrial pressures increase. It opposes the RAAS (shuts it off) Key Functions of ANP:

- Suppresses serum renin levels
- Decreases aldosterone release
- Increases glomerular filtration rate (excretion of Na+ and H2O)
- Decreases ADH release
- Decreases vascular resistance by causing vasodilation

MANAGEMENT OF HEART FAILURE

The primary goal of managing this condition is to improve LV function by:

- Decreasing intravascular volume
- Decreasing venous return
- Decreasing afterload
- Improving gas exchange and oxygenation
- Improving cardiac function
- Reducing anxiety

Nursing Management

Maintain airway, breathing, and circulation (ABCDE):

- Provide supplemental oxygen-High-flow oxygen (CPAP), (BiPAP) or administer oxygen therapy per nasal cannula at 2 - 6 LPM as ordered.

§ Heart Failure §

- RSI and ventilatory support for patients with respiratory compromise.
- Establish IV access for administration of crystalloid fluid/ medications, draw samples.
- Minimal fluid administration
- *Evaluate ABG analysis results:* semi-Fowler's or High-Fowler's position to promote greater lung expansion.
- *Promoting Rest and Activity:* Bed rest or limited activity may be necessary during the acute phase. Provide an overbed table close to the patient to allow resting the head and arms. Use pillows for added support when in High-Fowler's position.
  - Administer Diazepam (Valium) 2-10 mg 3 - 4 times a day as ordered to allay apprehension.
  - Gradual ambulation is encouraged to prevent risk of venous thrombosis and embolism due to prolonged immobility. Activities should progress through dangling, sitting up on a chair and then walking in increased distances under close supervision
  - Assess for signs of activity intolerance (dyspnea, fatigue and increased pulse rate that does not stabilize readily).
  - Decreasing Anxiety through:
    - ✓ Allow verbalization of feelings
    - ✓ Identify strengths that can be used for coping.
    - ✓ Learn what can be done to decrease anxiety.

§ Heart Failure §

Anxiety causes increased breathlessness which may be perceived by the client as an increase in the severity of the heart failure and this in turn increases anxiety.

- **Facilitating Fluid Balance through:**
  - ✓ Control of sodium intake
  - ✓ Administer diuretics and digitalis as prescribed
  - ✓ Monitor input and output, weight and V/S
  - ✓ Dry phlebotomy (rotating tourniquets)
- *Providing Skin Care.* Edematous skin is poorly nourished and susceptible to pressure sores. Prevent this through:
  - ✓ Change position at frequent intervals.
  - ✓ Assess the sacral area regularly.
  - ✓ Use protective devices to prevent pressure sores.
  - ✓ Promoting Nutrition. This is achieved through:
  - ✓ Provide bland, low-calorie, low residue with vitamin supplement during acute phase.
  - ✓ Frequent small feedings minimize exertion and reduce gastrointestinal blood requirements.
  - ✓ There may be no need to severely restrict sodium intake of the client who receives diuretics.
  - ✓ "No added salt" diet is prescribed. No processed foods in the diet.

♪ Heart Failure ♪

- **Promoting Elimination:**
  - ✓ Advise to avoid straining at defecation which involves Valsalva maneuver.
  - ✓ Administer laxative as ordered.
  - ✓ Encourage use of bedside commode.
- **Facilitating Learning:** Teach the client and his family about the disorder and self-care like:
  - ✓ Monitor signs and symptoms of recurring CHF (weight gain, loss of appetite, dyspnea, orthopnea, edema of the legs, persistent cough and report these to the physician).
  - ✓ Institute cardiac and pulse oximetry monitoring
  - ✓ Catheter placement and monitoring of pulmonary wedge and arterial pressures.
- Insert gastric tube and attach to suction if indicated Insert indwelling urinary catheter.
- *Monitoring:* Lab values: watching BNP, kidney function BUN and creatinine, troponins levels, electrolytes (especially potassium; if on Lasix there is wastage of potassium and low potassium increases risk of digoxin toxicity).
- **Edema in leg:** Keep legs elevated and patient in high Fowler's to help with breathing.
- **Safety** (at risk for falls due to fluid status changes, swelling in legs and feet, and orthostatic hypotension).

§ Heart Failure §

- Administer pharmacologic therapy as ordered: In administering medications, know the drug categories a patient will be taking with heart failure and what drugs are included in that category, the pharmacodynamics, and side effects. To remember the groups of drugs given, use the following mnemonic sentence:

'Always Administer Drugs Before A Ventricle Dies!'

Medical Management

ACE Inhibitors (Angiotensin Converting Enzyme Inhibitors):

These are the first line treatment for heart failure with beta blockers. They end in *"-pril"* e.g. Lisinopril, Ramipril, Enalapril, and Captopril.

These work by allowing more blood to get to the heart muscle which allows it to work easier. They also, block the conversion of Angiotensin I or Angiotensin II (this causes vasodilation, lowers blood pressure, and allows kidneys to secrete sodium because it decreases aldosterone).

Their side effects: dry, nagging cough and can increase potassium (inhibiting angiotensin II which decreases aldosterone in the body which causes the body to retain more potassium and excrete sodium).

§ Heart Failure §

ARBs (Angiotensin II Receptor Blockers):

They end in *"-sartan"* like Losartan, Valsartan used in place of ACE inhibitors if patient can't tolerate them blocks angiotensin II receptors which causes vasodilation. This lowers blood pressure and helps the kidneys to excrete sodium and water (due to the affects that blocking angiotensin II has on the kidneys; decreases aldosterone).

Their side effects: increases potassium levels, NO dry nagging cough. Used when the user fails to tolerate the ACEs.

Diuretics:

They are used along with ACE inhibitors or ARBs to decrease water and sodium retention which will decrease edema in the body and lungs. This allows the heart to pump easier.

Patients will urinate a lot! Loop diuretics (most common) like Lasix or Furosemide (watch potassium level because they will waste potassium). Potassium sparing diuretics like "Aldactone" (can cause hyperkalemia, especially if taking with ACE or ARBs).

Beta Blockers:

They block norepinephrine and epinephrine effects on the heart muscle given in stable heart failure with ACE inhibitors. They end in *"lol"* like Metoprolol, Carvedilol and Bisoprolol.

They are not used for acute heart failure because the negative inotropic effect on the heart. The negative inotropic effect causes decrease myocardial contractility (slows heart) and decreases

§ Heart Failure §

cardiac workload.

These drugs are used in stable heart failure in people with ventricular systolic dysfunction (there is a contraction problem with the left ventricle) and to treat diastolic heart failure (remember there is a problem with the heart filling in diastolic dysfunction). It will help the heart rest so the stiff ventricle can fill properly, and the volume of blood pumped out increases.

Their side effects: check pulse (bradycardia), no grape juice; mask hypoglycemic signs in diabetics, respiratory issues in asthmatics and patients with COPD.

Anticoagulants:

They are not used in all patients with heart failure. Typically, used in patients with heart failure who are in a-fib because they are at risk for blood clot formation or certain scenarios of left ventricular systolic heart failure when there is a low ejection fraction of <35%.

Vasodilators (arterial dilators):

Hydralazine prescribed with a nitrate like Isordil (venous dilator) sometimes used in place of an ACE or ARB, if patient can't tolerate them. This causes vasodilation in the arteries and veins to help decrease the amount of blood and fluid going back which helps decrease the workload on the heart.

Their side effects include low blood pressure, orthostatic

§ Heart Failure §

hypotension.

Digoxin

It is a positive inotropic effect that increases the heart's ability to contract stronger and it has a negative chronotropic action that causes the heart to beat slower. So, the heart slows down and contracts stronger which allows the heart to pump more blood.

They are used in treatment of patients with left ventricular systolic dysfunction (however, not usually the first line of treatment due to side effects and toxicity risks. It is used alongside ACE/beta blockers, and diuretics.

Toxicity issues: Monitor patient potassium level (hypokalemia <3.5 mEq/L) because hypokalemia increases digoxin toxicity.

Signs of toxicity: Nausea, vomiting, visual changes yellowish green halos. Check apical pulse before giving; >60 bpm. Its antidote is Digibind.

Angiotensin II receptor blockers (Losartan)

Amiodarone in arrhythmic patients

Bronchodilators

Given in patients with wheezing, "cardiac asthma."

Contraindicated Drugs in HF

NSAIDs: They worsen renal perfusion and reduce the effect of diuretics. They may trigger acute cardiac decompensation.

§ Heart Failure §

Calcium channel blockers (verapamil und diltiazem): They have a negative inotropic effect. They worsen symptoms and prognosis.

Thiazolidinediones: It promotes the progression of HF (increases fluid retention and edema) and increases the hospitalization rate.

Moxonidine: It increases mortality in HF with reduced ejection fraction (systolic dysfunction).

Trimethoprim-sulfamethoxazole: This causes hyperkalemia and inhibits the renal tubular creatinine secretion (reduced creatinine clearance). Significantly delayed excretion in chronic renal disease.

Invasive Procedures

Implantable cardiac defibrillator (ICD): This prevents sudden cardiac death. Primary prophylaxis indications of this include HF with EF < 35% and prior myocardial infarction/CHD, Increased risk of life-threatening cardiac arrhythmias. Secondary prophylaxis indications include history of sudden cardiac arrest, ventricular flutter, or ventricular fibrillation.

Cardiac Resynchronization Therapy (CRT): It improves cardiac function. Indicated in HF with EF < 35% and left bundle branch block. Can be combined with an ICD.

Coronary Revascularization with PCTA or Bypass Surgery: This may be indicated if CHD is present.

Valvular surgery if valvular heart defects are present.

Ventricular Assist Devices: a device that may be implanted to support ventricular function; may be indicated for temporary or long-term support (e.g., to bridge time until transplantation) of decompensated HF.

Cardiac transplantation: for patients with end-stage HF (NYHA class IV), ejection fraction < 20%, and no other viable treatment options.

MANAGEMENT OF ACUTE DECOMPENSATION OF HEART FAILURE

This is a sudden worsening of the signs and symptoms of heart failure, which typically includes difficulty breathing (dyspnea), leg or feet swelling, and fatigue. ADHF is a common and potentially serious cause of acute respiratory distress.

The condition is caused by severe congestion of multiple organs by fluid that is inadequately circulated by the failing heart. An attack of decompensation is usually caused by an underlying medical illness, such as myocardial infarction, an abnormal heart rhythm, infection, or thyroid disease.

It is therefore important to identify the precipitant of heart failure and treat it as the HF episode is being treated. The following is the regimen for the acute decompensated state of heart failure:

Diuretics

Lasix (Furosemide): Helps eliminate excess fluid that the heart cannot accommodate (preload) and improve stroke volume, thereby decreasing pulmonary and peripheral edema.

§ Heart Failure §

Morphine
Decreases preload by acting as a vasodilator and reduces sympathetic activation and consequently demand on heart by procuring pain relief.

Nitrates
Decrease preload via vasodilation and improve oxygen delivery to the heart.

Oxygen
Oxygen +/- noninvasive ventilation: preserve ventilator drive and maintaining blood oxygen saturation.

Positioning
Sit patient upright with legs dangling down to promote blood pooling in the lower extremities and decrease preload

Emergency Management of HF

HF can present acutely as acute HF or acute-on-chronic HF Acute HF. Usually the most prevalent clinical presentations are dyspnea, anxiety and tachycardia. Acute HF can evolve into cardiogenic shock, which is an acute circulatory failure due to improper/inappropriate fluid distribution.

Pallor and Hypotension (systolic <90), reduced CO and oliguria characterize cardiogenic shock.

§ Heart Failure §

Acute HF usually results from an acute event such as MI, arrhythmias, mechanical disease (valve rupture), pericardial disease e.t.c. Management involves:

- Sit up and start 100% oxygen flow
- Do an ECG, FBC, U/E, Cardiac enzymes, ABG, CXR
- Sublingual 2 puffs nitrates or oral to enhance myocardial perfusion.
- IV opiates (morphine 2.5-5mg) to reduce anxiety and preload
- IV furosemide 40-80mg I.V. to reduce fluid retention, hence pulmonary edema.
- If Systolic >90 then give IV infusion of isosorbide dinitrate 2-10mg/h, if Systolic <90 then treat as cardiogenic shock.
- In advanced situation can consider:
  - ✓ IV inotropic drug (dobutamine) to increase contractility and CO
  - ✓ IV Dopamine to enhance renal perfusion to prevent renal failure
  - ✓ IV aminophylline (slow infusion) to enhance contractility and bronchodilate.
  - ✓ Assisted ventilation

Modifiable Lifestyle Risk Factors

Lifestyle modification and patient education are paramount in

§ Heart Failure §

treating heart failure. This includes:
- Patient's personal needs and values must be considered
- Offer annual flu and a one-off pneumococcal vaccination.
- Smoking, alcohol, traveling, driving and sexual advice may be needed.
- *Exercise:* Involve in supervised physical activity as this increase general wellbeing.
- Diet: Increase in healthy food intake, reduce salt intake and monitor weight.
- Educating the early signs and symptoms heart failure exacerbation such as shortness of breath, weight gain and orthopnea.

Complications of Heart Failure

Some of the complications of heart failure include the following:
- Muscle under perfusion causing muscle weakness and atrophy causing fatigue, exercise intolerance and dyspnea.
- *Arrhythmias:* arrhythmias are tightly associated with HF and are responsible for a large proportion of death in patients with HF. Arrhythmias usually results from increase in fibrous tissue deposition during tissue remodeling post-insults. Arrhythmias themselves lead to HF therefore they worsen the situation when they exist.
- Increased risks of infections that can initiate an acute-on-

§ Heart Failure §

chronic event.
- Acute decompensated heart failure
- *Cardiorenal syndrome:* Cardiorenal syndrome is a complication of acute and chronic HF. This is a complex syndrome in which renal function progressively declines as a result of severe cardiac dysfunction. It occurs in about 20–30% of cases of acute decompensated HF. It happens in. Treat heart failure, manage renal failure to get rid of this situation.
- Central sleep apnea syndrome
- Cardiogenic shock
- *Stroke:* increased risk of arterial thromboembolisms (especially with concurrent atrial fibrillation).
- Chronic kidney disease
- Cardiac cirrhosis (congestive hepatopathy)
- Venous stasis, leg ulcers.

SUMMARY OF HEART FAILURE

Heart failure (HF) is a clinical condition in which the heart is unable to pump enough blood to meet the metabolic needs of the body because of pathological changes in the myocardium.

There are three main causes of HF and they include coronary heart disease, diabetes mellitus, and hypertension. These conditions cause ventricular dysfunction with low cardiac output, which results

§ Heart Failure §

in blood congestion (backward failure) and poor systemic perfusion (forward failure).

HF is classified as either left heart failure (LSHF) or right heart failure (RSHF), although biventricular HF is most commonly seen in in many seen cases.

LSHF leads to pulmonary edema and resulting dyspnea, while RHF induces systemic venous congestion that causes symptoms such as pitting edema, jugular venous distension, and hepatomegaly.

Biventricular HF manifests with clinical features of both RSHF and LSHF, as well as general symptoms such as tachycardia, fatigue, and nocturia. In rare cases, high-output HF may occur as a result of conditions that increase cardiac output and thereby overwhelm the heart.

Acute decompensated heart failure (ADHF) may occur as an exacerbation of HF or be caused by an acute cardiac condition such as myocardial infarction.

HF is diagnosed based on clinical presentation and requires an initial workup to assess disease severity and possible causes. Initial workup includes measurement of brain natriuretic peptide levels, chest x-ray, and an ECG.

Management of HF includes lifestyle modifications and treatment of associated conditions (e.g., hypertension) and comorbidities (e.g., anemia), along with pharmacologic agents that reduce the workload of the heart. ADHF requires hospitalization

§ Heart Failure §

and more intensive measures, such as hemodialysis.

2
~ RHEUMATIC FEVER ~

INTRODUCTION

The effects of rheumatic fever normally manifest in various parts of the body, but two major body systems are largely involved. The systems include the lymphatic (specifically immunity function) and the cardiovascular (specifically the heart which is mostly affected by the disease.

The latter has been covered in the first chapter) systems. The immune and the lymphatic systems work hand in hand in the provision of body's defense mechanisms in cases of skin or mucosal injuries, but more importantly during invasion by infectious agents.

THE PHYSIOLOGY OF BODY DEFENSE MECHANISMS

Non-Specific/Innate Immunity

This comprises of mechanical barriers that cover body surfaces (skin and mucous membranes), cells and chemicals that act in protecting the body from invading pathogens.

It responds immediately to protect the body from all foreign substances and also reduces the workload of the specific defense system by preventing entry and spread of micro-organisms throughout the body.

§ Rheumatic Fever §

There are many types of non-specific immunity in the body. One of the largest examples is the skin, which forms a tough, mechanical barrier that serves as the initial barrier to keep pathogens out of the body.

The skin cells actually secrete small proteins that destroy viruses as well. These barriers are grouped into two, body surface barriers and specialized cells. The body surface barriers include:

Physical Barriers

Include structures such as the skin and the mucous membranes of the body.

Chemical barriers which include:

- *Skin:* skin acidity (acid pH) inhibits bacterial growth and sebum is toxic to bacteria.
- *Stomach Mucosa:* it secretes HCL acid and protein-digesting enzymes that also have good protective effects on pathogens.
- *Oral cavity:* It contains saliva which consists of lysozyme that destroys bacteria as well.
- *Vagina:* secretions within it are highly acidic and they destroy bacteria.

Specialized cells

They protect the body from infectious agents in various ways. They include the following:

§ Rheumatic Fever §

- *Phagocytes:* Confronts pathogens that make it through the mechanical barriers in nearly everybody organ. They are of different types: macrophages, neutrophils.
- *Natural Killer (NK) Cells:* Unique group of defensive cells running in the blood stream and lymph that can lyse and kill cancer cells and virus-infected body cells before the immune system are enlisted in the fight.

Specific / Adaptive Immunity

Specific immunity, also known as adaptive immunity, is specialized immunity for particular pathogens. Helper T-cells, cytotoxic T-cells, and B-cells are involved in specific immunity. The non-specific cells, like macrophages, tell the T- and B-cells that an intruder is present.

The macrophages show the T- and B-cells parts of the pathogen, called antigens, so they know what to look for. Later, a special kind of cell called a memory cell creates a record of which intruders entered the body, so they can attack it faster during the next infection.

There are two types of specific T-cells: *helper T-cells* and *cytotoxic T-cells*. Helper T-cells recognize antigens from the macrophages and help to organize other cells in the immune system for a fight. Helper T-cells alert the rest of the immune system Helper T-cell.

Cytotoxic T-cells recognize infected cells and kill them before

§ Rheumatic Fever §

the infection spreads. They are like assassins, going in to kill the infected cells for the greater good. Even though the infected cells of the host die, the infection is contained, and damage is minimized.

In the following image, a host cell is letting a cytotoxic T-cell know it is infected by showing it the pathogen's antigen on the surface. The cytotoxic T-cell will then attach and destroy it.

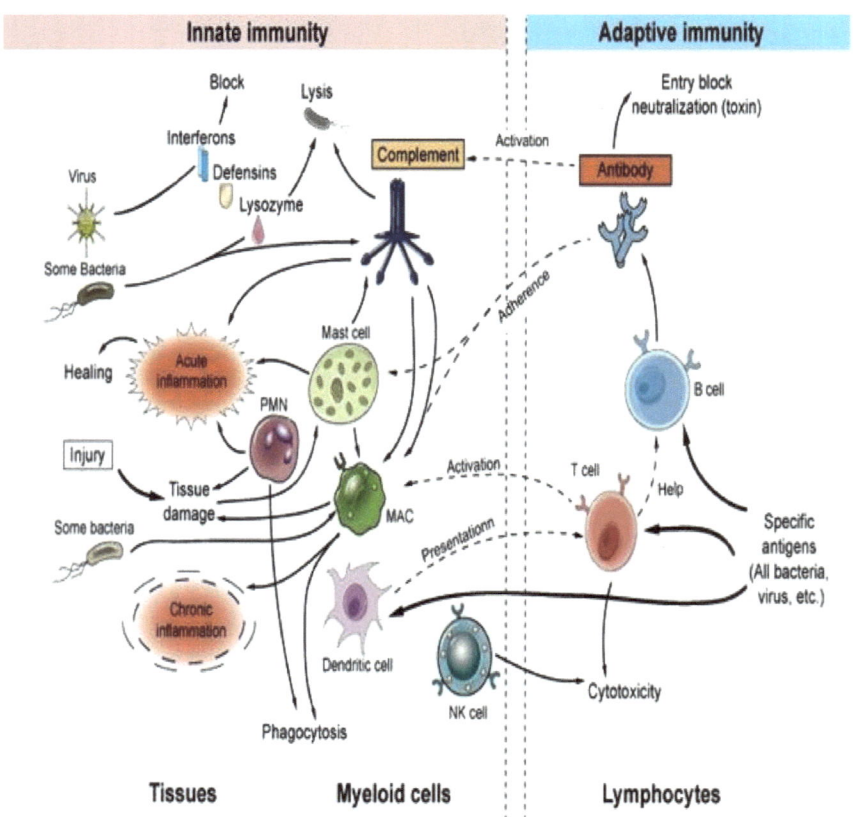

Activities of the Immune System Following an Attack

☙ Rheumatic Fever ❧

The Inflammatory Responses

When the body is first invaded by a bacterial infection, the purpose of the immune system is to control or eradicate it. The initial reaction of the immune system to an infection varies, depending on the site which has been invaded and on the nature of the invader. There can be many *"triggers"* that can spur the immune system into action.

Here are some of the ways in which the immune system can be activated. If the invasion is in an area of the body that is primarily defended by macrophages, such as the lungs or intestines, then these macrophages will be the first immune cells on the scene.

They begin to digest the invading organism, and by presenting antigens (proteins from the destroyed bacteria), they stimulate other cells of the immune system into action.

Some bacteria, for example Staphylococcus Aureus and Salmonella Typhi, produce chemotaxins when they enter the body, which betray their presence to the immune system, which reveal the location of the invader. Chemotaxins are chemicals that activate phagocytes, the immune cells whose function is to consume and destroy the invading bacteria.

The inflammatory response should only last for as long as the infection exists. Once the threat of infection has passed, the area should return to normal existence. Though, the actual process by which the inflammatory response ends is not well understood. The main symptoms of the inflammatory response are as follows:

§ Rheumatic Fever §

- The tissues in the area are red and warm, as a result of the large amount of blood reaching the site.
- The tissues in the area are swollen, again due to the increased amount of blood and proteins that are present.
- The area is painful, due the expansion of tissues, causing mechanical pressure on nerve cells, and also due to the presence of pain mediators.

Once the inflammatory process has begun, it continues until the infection that caused it has been eradicated. Phagocytes continue to consume and destroy bacteria, the acquired immune system binds and disposes of harmful toxins. Pus is then produced, pus being the debris that is left over from the battle between the invader and the immune system.

The colour of the pus depends on the organism causing the infection. Some bacteria first encounter, and are recognized by, the complement system, which in turn produces chemical messengers (cytokines) that warn other cells of the immune system that the body has been invaded.

The invader may be recognized by the acquired immune system, i.e. the lymphocytes. These cells either directly fight the infection themselves or control other cells to do so.

RHEUMATIC FEVER

Rheumatic fever (RF) also at times called or acute rheumatic fever (ARF) is an autoimmune inflammatory process that develops following a streptococcal infection. Rheumatic fever can involve the joints, skin, the brain and mostly the heart.

The disease typically develops two to four weeks after a streptococcal throat infection. The heart is involved in about half of the cases identified.

Damage to the heart valves by the infection leads to Rheumatic Heart Disease (RHD) usually occurring after repeated attacks of the infection but can sometimes occur after one episode. The damaged valves may result in heart failure, atrial fibrillation and infection of the valves.

Acute rheumatic fever (ARF) and its sequel, rheumatic heart disease (RHD), cause significant morbidity and mortality in developing countries, yet they are under-recognized as global health problems.

CAUSES OF RHEUMATIC FEVER

The main cause of RF is Group A streptococcus (GAS), a bacterium that can cause infections such as Strep throat with or without scarlet fever and skin infections like impetigo, and cellulitis. However, not all strains of streptococcal bacteria will lead to RF, and not everyone who has a GAS infection will develop RF.

Genetic factors may increase the risk. The chance of having RF appears to be higher if another family member has had it. The exact link between group A strep infection and RF remains unclear, but scientists believe that it is not the bacteria itself that causes the disease, but rather the immune system's faulty reaction to it. Strep bacteria have a protein that resembles one found in some body tissues.

Immune system cells that would usually target the bacteria may start attacking the body's own tissues instead, as if they are toxins or infectious agents. In RF, the tissues that they attack are those of the heart, joints, central nervous system (CNS) and skin.

These tissues react by becoming inflamed. If a patient with Strep bacteria takes a complete course of antibiotic treatment, the chances of RF developing are very low.

EPIDEMIOLOGY

Rheumatic fever occurs in about 325,000 children each year and about 33.4 million people currently have rheumatic heart disease. Those who develop RF are most often between the ages of 5 and 15, with 20% of first-time attacks occurring in adults. The disease is most common in the developing world and among indigenous peoples in the developed world.

In 2015 it resulted in 319,400 deaths down from 374,000 deaths in 1990. Most deaths occur in the developing world where as many as 12.5% of people affected may die each year.

RF incidences are similar in males and females but the risk of

§ Rheumatic Fever §

RHD is 1.6 – 2.0 times greater in women than men due to several factors including worsening of existing disease during pregnancy, GAS exposure during child rearing, limited access to services and intrinsic or hormonal factors.

The most recent estimates of the global burden of RHD alone include 9 million disability adjusted life years lost, 33 million prevalent cases and 275,000 deaths each year, with deaths occurring predominantly in low- and middle-income countries (LMICs).

RHD prevalence increases with age with survival varying with access and adherence to secondary prophylaxis to prevent ARF recurrence, severity of valvular damage and access to specialist management and surgery.

The epidemiology of RHD varies by region, with a particularly high prevalence in Africa and the Pacific region, but a high burden also in Latin America, the Middle East and Asia. The age distribution of prevalent RHD cases globally reflect two distinct epidemics. The first epidemic occurred until the mid-20th century in high-income countries where the majority of surviving prevalent cases is over 50 years of age with few incident cases.

The second on-going epidemic is characterized by a very high incidence in LMICs and among disadvantaged communities living in industrialized countries, such as minority indigenous peoples living in Australasia and North America.

This on-going epidemic is reflected in high proportions of cases at young ages, reducing with age due to poor survival. Australia is a good case study to contrast two populations experiencing different epidemics in the same country, using RHD/ARF hospital admission counts as a proxy for burden in Australia.

RHD is also associated with almost a quarter of prevalent Indigenous Australian stroke cases aged 20–34 years.

PATHOPHYSIOLOGY

Rheumatic fever is a late inflammatory, non-suppurative complication of pharyngitis that is caused by group A-hemolytic streptococci. Rheumatic fever results from humoral and cellular-mediated immune responses occurring 1-3 weeks after the onset of streptococcal pharyngitis.

Streptococcal proteins display molecular mimicry recognized by the immune system, especially bacterial M-proteins and human cardiac antigens such as myosin and valvular endothelium.

Antimyosin antibody recognizes laminin, an extracellular matrix alpha-helix coiled protein, which is part of the valve basement membrane structure. The valves most affected by rheumatic fever, in order, are the mitral, aortic, tricuspid, and pulmonary valves. In most cases, the mitral valve is involved with 1 or more of the other 3.

In acute disease, small thrombi form along the lines of valve closure. In chronic disease, there is thickening and fibrosis of the valve resulting in stenosis, or less commonly, regurgitation. T-cells that are responsive to the streptococcal M-protein infiltrate the valve through the valvular endothelium, activated by the binding of anti-streptococcal carbohydrates with release or tumor necrosis factor (TNF) and interleukins.

A study reported that the increased expression of Th17 cell-associated cytokines might play an important role in the pathogenesis and development of rheumatic heart disease.

The acute involvement of the heart in rheumatic fever gives rise to pancarditis, with inflammation of the myocardium, pericardium, and endocardium.

Carditis occurs in approximately 40-50% of patients on the first attack; however, the severity of acute carditis has been questioned. Pericarditis occurs in 5-10% of patients with rheumatic fever; isolated myocarditis is rare.

CLINICAL PRESENTATIONS

Symptoms of strep throat include:
- Sore throat
- Headache
- Swollen, tender lymph nodes
- Trouble swallowing
- Nausea and vomiting
- Red skin rash
- High temperature
- Swollen tonsils

⸹ Rheumatic Fever ⸹

- Abdominal pain

Signs and symptoms generally develop 2 to 4 weeks after a streptococcal infection. Some individuals will experience just one or two of the following symptoms, but others may experience most of them:

- Fatigue
- Rapid heart rate
- Decreased ability to exercise
- Joint pain and swelling
- Fever
- Plotchy rash
- Uncontrollable twitching and movements

Arthritis, or pain and swelling in the joints, affects 75 percent of patients. It normally starts in the larger joints, such as the knees, ankles, wrists, and elbows, before moving to other joints. This inflammation normally resolves within 4-6 weeks, without causing permanent damage.

The heart accounts for 30–60% of cases. Inflammation of the heart can lead to chest pain, palpitations, a sensation that the heart is fluttering or pounding hard, panting, and shortness of breath, and fatigue. Other heart symptoms include:

- Pancarditis (endocarditis, myocarditis, and pericarditis)
- Valvular lesions:
  - ✓ Early mitral regurgitation or prolapse
- Late mitral stenosis: Rheumatic fever is the most

§ Rheumatic Fever §

frequent cause of mitral stenosis.
- Mixed mitral stenosis/regurgitation also possible
- Aortic valve (25% of cases)
- Aortic regurgitation
- Aortic stenosis
- Tricuspid valve (10% of cases)

Dilated cardiomyopathy due to severe valvular disease, myocarditis.

CNS manifestations (up to 25% of cases). Some of the signs are as follows:

- *Sydenham Chorea*: Occurs 1–8 months after the inciting infection. It is involuntary, irregular, non-repetitive movements of the limbs, neck, head, and/or face, sometimes asymmetrical or confined to one side (hemichorea).
- Additional motor symptoms such as ballismus, muscle weakness) and speech disorders (slurred or "jerky" speech).
- Neuropsychiatric symptoms such as inappropriate laughing/crying, agitation, anxiety, apathy, obsessive-compulsive behavior.
- Skin (up to 10% of cases), it includes features such as:
  - Subcutaneous Nodules
  - *Erythema Marginatum*: centrifugally expanding pink or light red rash with a well- defined outer border (erythema marginatum; marginated rash) and central

§ Rheumatic Fever §

clearing.

They are normally located at the trunk and limbs are affected; the face is spared. May rapidly appear and disappear at different locations. They are painless and non-pruritic

DIAGNOSIS

History and physical examination for the presence of strep infection and other features.

Jones Criteria for RF diagnosis: Modified Jones criteria was first published in 1944 by T. Duckett Jones, MD. It has periodically been revised by the American Heart Association in collaboration with other groups.

According to revised Jones criteria, the diagnosis of rheumatic fever can be made when two of the *major criteria*, or one major criterion plus two *minor criteria*, are present along with evidence of streptococcal infection. The criteria are as follows:

Major Criteria

This includes the following:

- *Polyarthritis:* A temporary migrating inflammation of the large joints, usually starting in the legs and migrating upwards.
- *Carditis:* Inflammation of the heart muscle (myocarditis) which can manifest as congestive heart failure with shortness of breath, pericarditis with a rub, or a new heart

murmur.
- *Subcutaneous nodules:* These are painless, firm collections of collagen fibers over bones or tendons. They commonly appear on the back of the wrist, the outside elbow, and the front of the knees.
- *Erythema marginatum:* A long-lasting reddish rash that begins on the trunk or arms as macules, which spread outward and clear in the middle to form rings, which continue to spread and coalesce with other rings, ultimately taking on a snake-like appearance. This rash typically spares the face and is made worse with heat.
- *Sydenham's chorea (St. Vitus' Dance):* A characteristic series of involuntary rapid movements of the face and arms. This can occur very late in the disease for at least three months from onset of infection.

Minor Criteria
This includes the following:
- Fever of 38.2–38.9 °C (100.8–102.0 °F)
- *Arthralgia:* Joint pain without swelling (Cannot be included if polyarthritis is present as a major symptom).
- Raised erythrocyte sedimentation rate or C reactive protein.
- Leukocytosis

ECG showing features of heart block, such as a prolonged PR

§ Rheumatic Fever §

interval (Cannot be included if carditis is present as a major symptom). Previous episode of rheumatic fever or inactive heart disease.

Other tests may include the following:

- *Echocardiogram (ECHO):* This test uses sound waves to check the heart's chambers and valves. The echo sound waves create a picture on a screen as an ultrasound transducer is passed over the skin overlying the heart. Echo can show damage to the valve flaps, backflow of blood through a leaky valve, fluid around the heart, and heart enlargement. It's the most useful test for diagnosing heart valve problems.
- *Electrocardiogram (ECG):* This test records the strength and timing of the electrical activity of the heart. It shows abnormal rhythms (arrhythmias or dysrhythmias) and can sometimes detect heart muscle damage. Small sensors are taped to your skin to pick up the electrical activity.
- *Chest X-ray:* An X-ray may be done to check your lungs and see if your heart is enlarged.
- *Cardiac MRI:* This is an imaging test that takes detailed pictures of the heart. It may be used to get a more precise look at the heart valves and heart muscle.
- *Blood tests:* Certain blood tests may be used to look for infection and inflammation. For example, blood culture and full hemogram.

Rheumatic Fever

MANAGEMENT OF RHEUMATIC FEVER

Treatment strategies for acute rheumatic fever (ARF) can be divided into the following:

- Management of the acute attack
- Management of the current infection
- Prevention of further infection and attacks

The primary goal of treating an ARF attack is to eradicate streptococcal organisms and bacterial antigens from the pharyngeal region.

Penicillin is the drug of choice in persons who are not at risk of allergic reaction. A single of an injection of benzathine penicillin can ensure compliance.

The American Heart Association (AHA) Committee on Acute Rheumatic Fever recommends a regimen consisting of benzathine benzylpenicillin at 1.2 million units intramuscularly every 4 weeks. However, in high-risk situations, administration every 3 weeks is justified and advised.

Oral cephalosporins, rather than erythromycin, are also recommended as an alternative in patients who are allergic to penicillin.

Prompt treatment of streptococcal pharyngitis in susceptible hosts can prevent repetitive exposure to pathologically reactive antigens.

However, management of the current infection will probably not affect the course of the current attack. Antimicrobial therapy does not alter the course, frequency, or severity of cardiac involvement.

Analgesia is optimally achieved with high doses of salicylates, which often induce dramatic clinical improvement. However, a lower dose may be required to avert symptoms of nausea and vomiting.

When *salicylates* are used as therapy, the dosage should be increased until the drug produces either a clinical effect or systemic toxicity characterized by tinnitus, headache, or hyperpnoea.

Corticosteroids should be reserved for the treatment of severe carditis. After 2-3 weeks, the dosage may be tapered, reduced by 25% each week. Overlap with high-dose salicylate therapy is recommended as the dosage of the prednisone is tapered over a 2-week period to avoid post steroid rebound. In extreme cases, intravenous methylprednisolone may be used.

Mild heart failure usually responds to rest and corticosteroid therapy. Digoxin can be useful in patients with severe carditis, but its use should be monitored closely because of the possibility of heart block.

Nocturnal tachycardia may be a sign of cardiac involvement that may be responsive to digoxin. Vasodilators and diuretics also may be used.

Sydenham chorea requires long-term antimicrobial prophylaxis, even if no other manifestations of rheumatic fever evolve. A number of drugs have been used off label for symptomatic treatment of Sydenham chorea, including anticonvulsants (e.g., valproate, carbamazepine) and neuroleptics (e.g., pimozide, haloperidol, risperidone, and olanzapine).

In underdeveloped countries, prophylaxis should be continued as follows:
- Continue for 5 years after the first attack
- Continue indefinitely in patients with established heart disease
- Continue indefinitely in patients who are frequently exposed to streptococci and are difficult to monitor

Surgical Care: Valve replacement should be considered in patients with active carditis, especially those with cases that are refractory to medical care or require high doses of vasodilators and diuretics.

Regurgitant lesions respond to valve replacement. Pure stenotic lesions may benefit from more conservative balloon mitral commissurotomy.

COMPLICATIONS OF RHEUMATIC FEVER

Rheumatic heart disease is a major complication of RF. Presence of this; the patient can develop the following:

Heart failure

The major cause of death and disability from RHD is heart failure. Over time, scarred and damaged heart valves make it impossible

§ Rheumatic Fever §

for the heart to pump blood effectively. Without a well-functioning heart, fluid builds up in the lungs and body, causing symptoms like breathlessness, swelling and fatigue. These symptoms tend to become worse over time without treatment.

🞣 Stroke

A *'stroke'* occurs when a part of the brain does not receive adequate blood supply. Strokes can be from clot which blocks a blood vessel (ischemic) or from a burst blood vessel (hemorrhagic). People with RHD are at risk of ischemic stroke because of blood clots which can form in the heart and subsequently block blood flow to parts of the brain.

🞣 Arrhythmias

Atrial fibrillation (AF) is an abnormal heart rhythm. People with RHD are at risk of AF because heart valve damage changes the shape of the heart and increased the risk of AF. AF tends to make heart failure worse, increasing shortness of breath, and may cause palpitations.

🞣 Endocarditis

Infective endocarditis (IE) is a bacterial infection on the valves of the heart. Valves that are already scarred or damaged by RHD are more likely to have IE than undamaged valves. People with IE have fevers and the heart may be unable to pump blood effectively.

§ Rheumatic Fever §

🞣 Complications in pregnancy

Women with RHD are at risk of significant illness or death during pregnancy and labour. The changes of pregnancy make the heart work harder. Hearts that have been damaged by RHD may not be able to adjust to these changes causing heart failure. The symptoms of heart failure may be confused with symptoms of late pregnancy and go untreated, causing cardiovascular collapse and death.

PREVENTION

Primary prevention

It includes prompt antibiotic treatment (e.g., penicillins) of GAS tonsillopharyngitis diagnosed by throat culture or rapid strep test.

Secondary prevention

Antibiotic prophylaxis to prevent recurrence and the drug of choice is IM penicillin G benzathine. In patients with a penicillin allergy, oral macrolides immediately follow antibiotic treatment of acute rheumatic fever. The duration depends on risk and severity of original episode.

Rheumatic fever without carditis

5 years or until the patient is age 21 (whichever is longer).

§ Rheumatic Fever §

Rheumatic fever with carditis

10 years or until the patient is age 21 (whichever is longer). Rheumatic fever with carditis and permanent valvular heart defects: 10 years or until age 40 (whichever is longer).

SUMMARY

Rheumatic fever is caused by an autoimmune response to throat infection with Streptococcus pyogenes. Cardiac involvement during rheumatic fever attack can result in rheumatic heart disease, which can cause heart failure and premature death.

Poverty and household overcrowding are associated with an increased prevalence of rheumatic fever and rheumatic heart disease, both of which remain a public health problem in many low-income countries.

Control efforts are hampered by the scarcity of accurate data on disease burden, and effective approaches to diagnosis, prevention, and treatment.

The diagnosis of rheumatic fever is entirely clinical, without any laboratory gold standard, and no treatments have been shown to reduce progression to rheumatic heart disease.

Prevention mainly relies on the prompt recognition and treatment of streptococcal pharyngitis, and avoidance of recurrent infection using long-term antibiotics (Penicillins), but evidence for the effectiveness of either approach is not strong.

More intensive studies are needed to provide the needed

§ Rheumatic Fever §

guidance to reduce rheumatic fever incidences and prevent its progression into rheumatic heart disease.

REFERENCES

Kawai T. and Akira S. (2006). "Innate immune recognition of viral infection". *Nature Immunology.* 7 (2): 131–7.

Middleton D, Curran M. and Maxwell L. (2002). "Natural killer cells and their receptors". *Transplant Immunology.* 10 (2–3): 147–64.

Phibbs, Brendan (2007). *The human heart: a basic guide to heart disease (2nd ed.).* Philadelphia: Lippincott Williams & Wilkins.

State University of New York (2014). "The Circulatory System." Suny.edu. *Archived from the original on February 3, 2014.*

"Suffering has been stronger than all other teaching and has taught me to understand what your heart used to be. I have been bent and broken, but - I hope - into a better shape."

~ *From 'Great Expectations' by Charles Dickens*

~ THE END ~

Ishmael Onserio

www.ingramcontent.com/pod-product-compliance
Lightning Source LLC
Chambersburg PA
CBHW040223220526
45473CB00001B/104